Low FODMAP Diet Cookbook

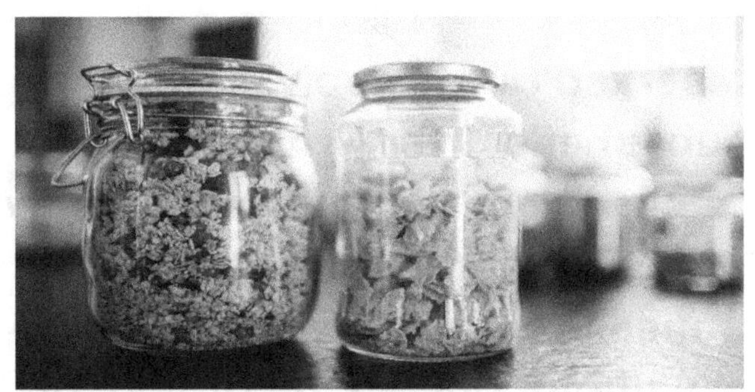

Take Charge of IBS and other Digestive Disorder with These Easy and Fast Mouthwatering Recipes

VICKIE CLARK

TABLE OF CONTENT

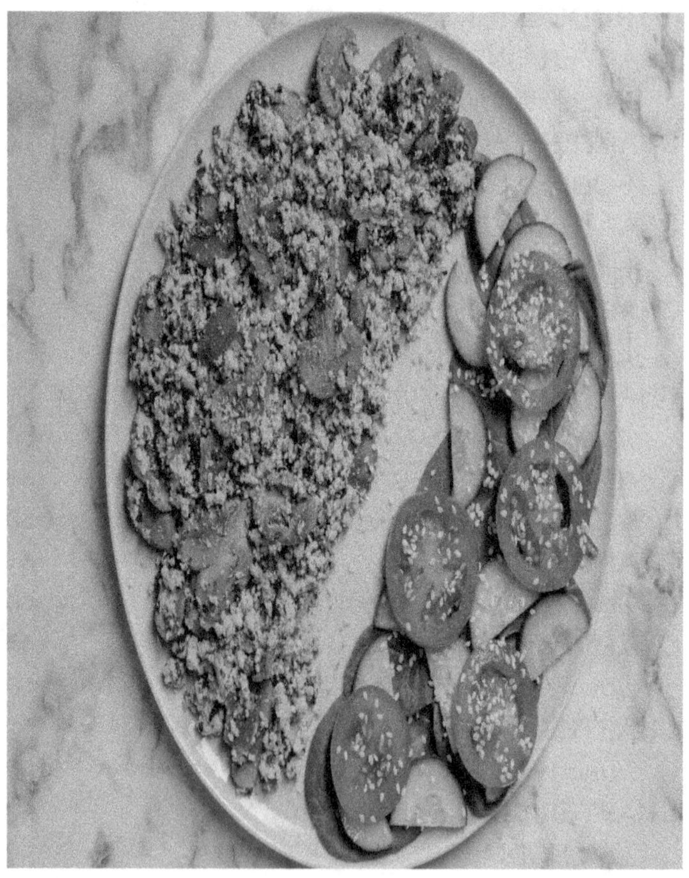

INTRODUCTION

The low FODMAP diet cookbook offers a comprehensive guide to managing symptoms of irritable bowel syndrome (IBS) and other gastrointestinal disorders. FODMAPs, fermentable oligosaccharides, disaccharides, monosaccharides, and polyols, are a group of carbohydrates that can trigger digestive discomfort in some individuals. This cookbook introduces readers to the low FODMAP diet, which involves reducing intake of these fermentable carbohydrates to alleviate symptoms such as bloating, gas, abdominal pain, and diarrhea. include information on who might benefit from following the diet, such as individuals with IBS, inflammatory bowel disease (IBD), small intestinal bacterial overgrowth (SIBO), or other functional gastrointestinal disorders.

Furthermore, the introduction usually outlines the three main phases of the low FODMAP diet: elimination, reintroduction, and maintenance. During the elimination phase, high FODMAP foods are avoided to help identify trigger foods. The reintroduction phase involves systematically reintroducing FODMAPs to determine individual tolerance levels. Finally, the maintenance phase focuses on long-term dietary management, where individuals can enjoy a varied diet while minimizing symptoms.

Additionally, the introduction may provide tips for success on the low FODMAP diet, such as working with a healthcare professional or registered dietitian, reading food labels carefully, and planning meals ahead of time. It may also address common challenges and misconceptions about the diet, as well as potential nutrient concerns and how to ensure a balanced diet while following low FODMAP guidelines.

Overall, the introduction sets the stage for the recipes and resources provided in the cookbook, empowering readers to take control of their digestive health through mindful and delicious eating choices.

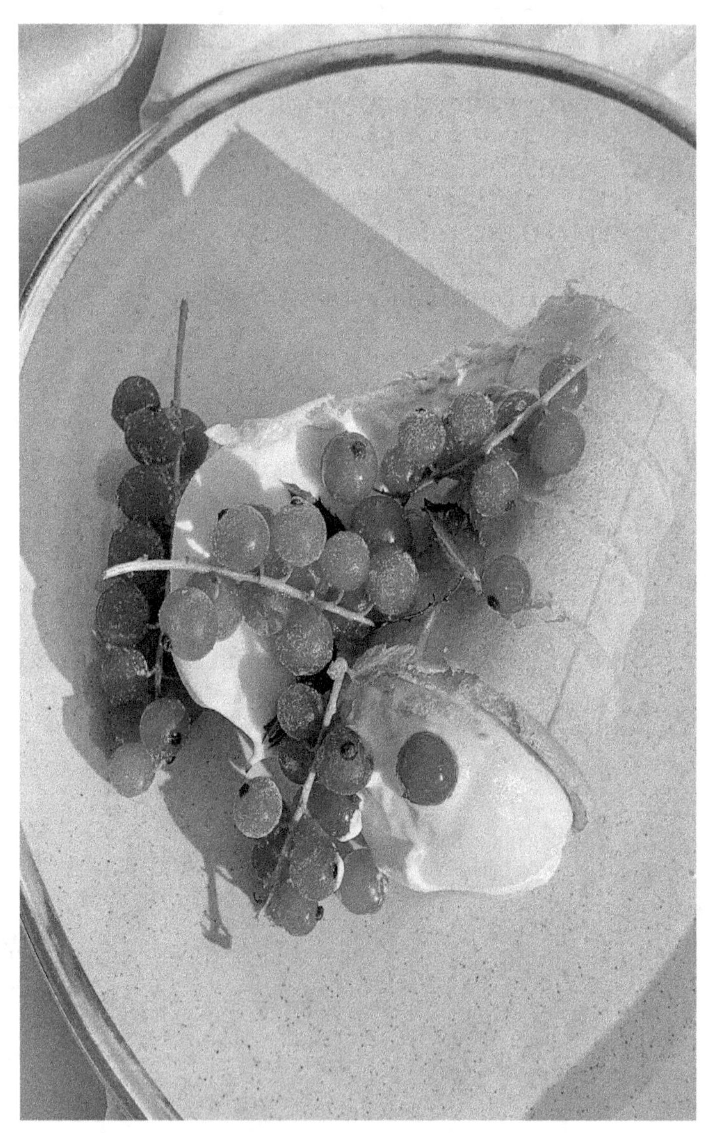

CHAPTER ONE

Understanding FODMAPS And IBS

FODMAPs are an acronym for monosaccharides, polyols, disaccharides, and fermentable oligosaccharides. They are a group of short-chain carbohydrates (sugars) that are poorly absorbed in the small intestine and can ferment in the colon. This fermentation process can lead to gas, bloating, abdominal pain, and other gastrointestinal symptoms in some people, particularly those with irritable bowel syndrome (IBS) or other digestive disorders.

The types of FODMAPs include:

1. ***Algae consisting of short chains of sugar molecules are called oligosaccharides***. The main types of oligosaccharides found in foods are fructans and galacto-oligosaccharides (GOS). Foods high in oligosaccharides include wheat, rye, onions, garlic, legumes, and certain fruits like watermelon and apples.

2. ***Disaccharides***: These are double sugar molecules. The primary disaccharide in the diet is lactose, found in dairy products such as milk, cheese, and yogurt.

3. ***Monosaccharides***: These are single sugar molecules. The monosaccharide of concern in the FODMAP diet is fructose, particularly when consumed in excess of glucose. Foods high in

fructose include certain fruits like apples, pears, mangoes, and honey.

4. ***Polyols***: Also known as sugar alcohols, polyols are found naturally in some fruits and vegetables and are used as artificial sweeteners in sugar-free gums and candies. Sorbitol, mannitol, xylitol, and maltitol are examples of common polyols. Foods high in polyols include certain fruits like cherries, plums, and peaches, as well as some vegetables like cauliflower and mushrooms.

The low FODMAP diet is an approach used to manage symptoms associated with conditions such as IBS. It involves restricting foods high in FODMAPs for a period of time, typically 2-6 weeks, followed by a structured reintroduction phase to identify individual triggers. During the elimination phase, foods high in FODMAPs are limited to reduce symptoms, and then gradually reintroduced to determine which specific FODMAPs trigger symptoms in each person.

It's important to note that the low FODMAP diet is not a lifelong diet but rather a temporary approach to identify and manage triggers for gastrointestinal symptoms. It should be undertaken with the guidance of a healthcare professional or registered dietitian to ensure nutritional adequacy and proper implementation. Additionally, not everyone with digestive issues will benefit from a low FODMAP diet, so individualized assessment and recommendations are key.

CHAPTER TWO

FODMAPS Digestion Difficulty

FODMAPs, which stands for Fermentable Oligosaccharides, Disaccharides, Monosaccharides, and Polyols, are a group of short-chain carbohydrates and sugar alcohols found in many foods. While they are generally considered healthy, they can be difficult to digest for some people, particularly those with certain gastrointestinal conditions like irritable bowel syndrome (IBS). Here are several reasons why FODMAPs can be challenging to digest:

1. *Poor Absorption*: FODMAPs are small molecules that are not well absorbed in the small intestine. This can lead to

them passing into the large intestine relatively intact, where they can ferment and cause gastrointestinal symptoms like bloating, gas, and discomfort.

2. ***Osmotic Effect***: Some FODMAPs have an osmotic effect, meaning they draw water into the intestine. This can lead to diarrhea, especially in individuals who are sensitive to these compounds.

3. ***Fermentation:*** In the large intestine, FODMAPs are fermented by bacteria. This fermentation process produces gasses like hydrogen, methane, and carbon dioxide, which can cause bloating, flatulence, and abdominal pain.

4. ***Individual Variability***: Not everyone has the same level of difficulty digesting FODMAPs. Some people may be able to tolerate certain FODMAPs better than

others, while others may have a heightened sensitivity to even small amounts.

5. ***Fructose Malabsorption***: Fructose, a monosaccharide found in fruits and some sweeteners, can be challenging to digest for some individuals, especially when consumed in excess of glucose. This can lead to symptoms like bloating, abdominal pain, and diarrhea.

6. ***Lactose Intolerance:*** Lactose, a disaccharide found in dairy products, can be difficult to digest for individuals who are lactose intolerant, meaning they lack the enzyme lactase needed to break it down. This can lead to symptoms like bloating, gas, and diarrhea after consuming lactose-containing foods.

7. ***Polyols****:* Polyols, or sugar alcohols, are found in certain fruits and vegetables as well as some artificial sweeteners. They are poorly absorbed in the small intestine and can ferment in the large intestine, leading to gastrointestinal symptoms in susceptible individuals.

8. ***FODMAP-Rich Foods:*** Many healthy foods are rich in FODMAPs, including fruits like apples and pears, vegetables like onions and garlic, legumes, wheat products, and certain dairy products. For individuals with digestive issues, avoiding or limiting these foods can be challenging, as they may need to carefully manage their diet to minimize symptoms.

In summary, FODMAPs can be difficult to digest due to their poor absorption, osmotic effect, fermentation by gut bacteria, individual variability in tolerance, and the presence of specific types of carbohydrates and sugar alcohols in certain foods. Managing intake of FODMAP-containing foods may be necessary for individuals with gastrointestinal conditions like IBS to reduce symptoms and improve quality of life.

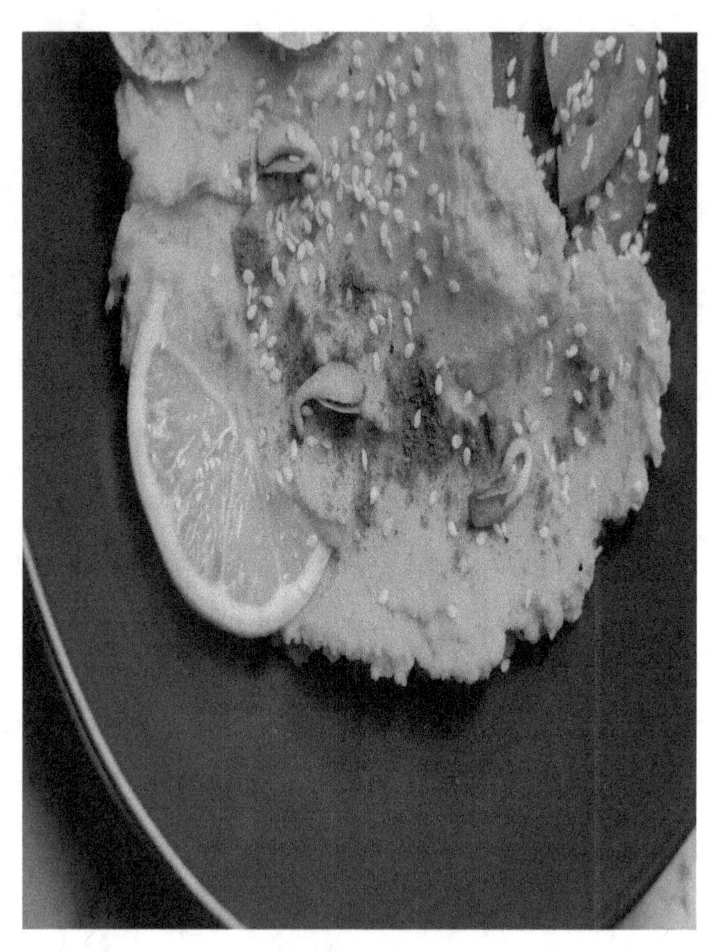

CHAPTER THREE

High FODMAPS Food

A class of short-chain carbohydrates and sugar alcohols known as FODMAPs (Fermentable Oligosaccharides, Disaccharides, Monosaccharides, and Polyols) are poorly absorbed in the small intestine. For people with certain digestive disorders like irritable bowel syndrome (IBS) or functional gastrointestinal disorders (FGIDs), consuming high-FODMAP foods can lead to symptoms such as bloating, gas, abdominal pain, and diarrhea.

Here's an extensive list of foods that are high in FODMAPs:

1. Fruits:

- o Apples
- o Pears
- o Watermelon
- o Cherries
- o Mangoes
- o Nectarines
- o Peaches
- o Plums
- o Rambutan
- o Lychee
- o Blackberries
- o Apricots
- o Tinned fruit in natural juice containing apple or pear juice concentrate

2. *Vegetables:*
   - o Onions (all types)
   - o Garlic
   - o Shallots

- Leeks
- Artichokes (globes, Jerusalem)
- Asparagus
- Beetroot
- Cauliflower
- Mushrooms
- Snow peas
- Sugar snap peas

3. *Legumes and Pulses:*

- Beans (kidney, black-eyed peas, butter, chickpeas)
- Lentils
- Peas (green, black-eyed)

4. *Dairy Products:*

- Cow's milk
- Soft cheeses (e.g., ricotta, cottage cheese)
- Cream
- Custard

o Yogurt with added sweeteners

5. Grains:

o Wheat-based products (bread, pasta, couscous)

o Barley

o Rye

o Some types of breakfast cereals

o Foods containing wheat-derived ingredients like wheat dextrin or wheat starch

6. Sweeteners:

o Honey

o High-fructose corn syrup

o Sorbitol

o Mannitol

o Xylitol

o Isomalt

7. Miscellaneous:

- ○ Certain alcoholic beverages (beer, some fortified wines)
- ○ Certain nuts and seeds (cashews, pistachios)
- ○ Some processed foods with high FODMAP ingredients

It's important to note that FODMAP sensitivity can vary among individuals, and some people may be able to tolerate small amounts of certain high-FODMAP foods without experiencing symptoms. However, for those following a low-FODMAP diet under the guidance of a healthcare professional, it's generally advised to avoid or limit these foods to manage symptoms effectively.

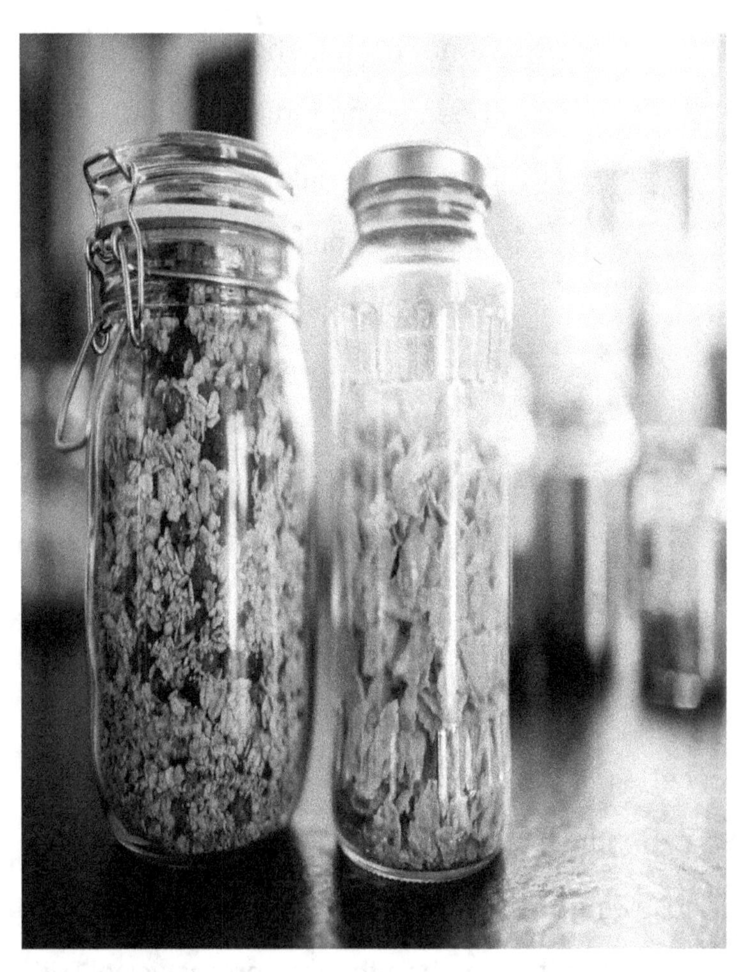

CHAPTER FOUR

Low FODMAPS Overview

Low FODMAPs (Fermentable Oligosaccharides, Disaccharides, Monosaccharides, and Polyols) diet is a dietary approach designed to manage symptoms of irritable bowel syndrome (IBS) and other functional gastrointestinal disorders (FGIDs) by reducing the consumption of specific carbs that are not well absorbed in the small intestine. These carbohydrates, when fermented by gut bacteria, can produce gas and other uncomfortable symptoms such as bloating, abdominal pain, and altered bowel habits in sensitive individuals.

Here's a comprehensive overview of low FODMAPs foods:

1. *What are FODMAPs?*

- FODMAPs are short-chain carbohydrates that are resistant to digestion and absorption in the small intestine.
- They can be categorized into five groups:
  - Oligosaccharides: Found in foods like wheat, rye, onions, garlic, legumes, and some fruits.
  - Disaccharides: Lactose, which is present in dairy products such as soft cheeses, yogurt, and milk.
  - Monosaccharides: Fructose, found in fruits like apples, pears, mangoes, and honey.

- **Polyols:** Sugar alcohols like sorbitol, mannitol, xylitol, and maltitol, found in certain fruits and vegetables and used as artificial sweeteners.

- **(And)** And stands for And More, which refers to other types of carbohydrates that may also cause digestive discomfort in some individuals.

2. ***Low FODMAPs Diet*:**

- Developed by researchers at Monash University, the low FODMAPs diet involves restricting high-FODMAP foods for a certain period, followed by systematic reintroduction to identify specific triggers.

- It's typically divided into three phases: elimination, reintroduction, and maintenance.
- The elimination phase involves avoiding high-FODMAP foods for a few weeks to alleviate symptoms.
- During the reintroduction phase, foods are systematically reintroduced in small amounts to identify personal triggers.
- The maintenance phase involves a personalized diet plan that minimizes symptoms by avoiding high-FODMAP foods while maximizing nutritional variety.

3. *Low FODMAPs Foods:*

- Low FODMAPs foods include:

    - Proteins: Meat, poultry, fish, eggs, tofu.

    - Grains: Rice, oats, quinoa, corn.

    - Fruits: Berries (strawberries, blueberries, raspberries), citrus fruits (oranges, lemons, limes), bananas, grapes.

    - Vegetables: Leafy greens (spinach, kale, lettuce), carrots, bell peppers, cucumber, zucchini, potatoes (small portions), tomatoes.

    - Almond milk, coconut milk, lactose-free yogurt, and

lactose-free milk are dairy substitutes.

- Fats and oils: Olive oil, coconut oil, butter.
- Nuts and seeds: Almonds (in small portions), peanuts, pumpkin seeds, sunflower seeds.

- It's essential to pay attention to portion sizes, as some low FODMAPs foods can become high FODMAPs in larger quantities.

4. Meal Planning:

- Creating balanced meals on a low FODMAPs diet involves combining low FODMAPs foods from different food groups to ensure adequate nutrition.

- This may include incorporating protein sources, carbohydrates from low FODMAPs grains and vegetables, healthy fats, and suitable snacks.
- Planning ahead and experimenting with recipes can help maintain variety and enjoyment in the diet while avoiding high FODMAPs triggers.

5. **Considerations:**

- While the low FODMAPs diet can be effective in managing IBS symptoms, it's essential to work with a healthcare professional or registered dietitian to ensure nutritional adequacy and proper implementation.

- The diet may not be suitable for everyone, and individual tolerance to specific FODMAPs may vary.
- Additionally, the diet is not intended for long-term use but rather as a short-term intervention to identify and manage triggers.

Overall, the low FODMAPs diet can be a valuable tool for individuals with IBS or FGIDs in managing their symptoms and improving their quality of life, but it should be carried out under the supervision of a medical professional to guarantee security and efficacy.

CHAPTER FIVE

Low FODMAPS Diet Basics

The low FODMAP diet is a dietary approach primarily used to manage symptoms of irritable bowel syndrome (IBS), a common gastrointestinal disorder. FODMAPs are fermentable oligosaccharides, disaccharides, monosaccharides, and polyols, which are types of carbohydrates that are poorly absorbed in the small intestine. When FODMAPs reach the large intestine, they ferment and draw water into the colon, leading to symptoms such as bloating, gas, abdominal pain, and diarrhea in susceptible individuals.

The low FODMAP diet works by reducing the intake of these fermentable carbohydrates, thereby decreasing their fermentation in the gut and alleviating symptoms associated with IBS. Here's how it typically works:

1. ***Elimination Phase:*** During this phase, high FODMAP foods are eliminated from the diet for a period of usually 2-6 weeks. Common high FODMAP foods include certain fruits (e.g., apples, cherries), vegetables (e.g., onions, garlic), legumes (e.g., beans, lentils), dairy products containing lactose, wheat products, and sweeteners like sorbitol and mannitol. This phase helps to identify which FODMAPs trigger symptoms in an individual.

2. ***Reintroduction Phase:*** After the elimination phase, FODMAP-containing foods are systematically reintroduced into the diet one at a time, in small

amounts, to identify specific triggers. This phase helps to determine which FODMAPs are well-tolerated and which ones exacerbate symptoms.

3. ***Personalization Phase:*** Based on the individual's tolerance levels identified during the reintroduction phase, a personalized long-term diet plan is developed. This phase aims to maintain a diet that minimizes symptoms while providing adequate nutrition.

4. ***Monitoring and Maintenance:*** After establishing a personalized diet plan, ongoing monitoring and occasional adjustments may be necessary to ensure symptom management and nutritional adequacy.

The low FODMAP diet is not a one-size-fits-all approach, and it's essential to work with a healthcare professional, such as a registered dietitian, throughout the process. They can provide guidance on implementing the diet, ensure nutritional needs are met, and offer support for long-term management of IBS symptoms. Additionally, it's important to note that the low FODMAP diet is not meant to be followed strictly for the long term but rather to identify trigger foods and establish a sustainable eating pattern that minimizes symptoms.

CHAPTER SIX

Low FODMAPS Diet Benefits

The low FODMAP diet is a dietary approach designed to help manage symptoms of irritable bowel syndrome (IBS) and other gastrointestinal disorders. FODMAPs stands for Fermentable Oligosaccharides, Disaccharides, Monosaccharides, and Polyols, which are types of carbohydrates that are poorly absorbed in the small intestine and can ferment in the colon, leading to symptoms like bloating, gas, abdominal pain, and diarrhea in some individuals. The following are a few advantages of eating a low-FODMAPS diet:

1. ***Symptom Relief for IBS***: One of the primary benefits of the low FODMAP diet is its effectiveness in reducing symptoms of IBS, such as bloating, gas, abdominal pain, and diarrhea. Research has shown that up to 75% of people with IBS experience symptom improvement when following a low FODMAP diet.

2. ***Customized Approach***: There is no one-size-fits-all strategy when it comes to the low-FODMAPS diet. The procedure entails removing and reintroducing foods to determine which ones are trigger foods for each individual. This personalized approach allows people to tailor their diet to their own sensitivities and preferences.

3. ***Improved Quality of Life:*** By reducing or eliminating symptoms of IBS, the low

FODMAP diet can significantly improve quality of life for those who suffer from gastrointestinal discomfort. It allows individuals to enjoy meals without fear of triggering unpleasant symptoms.

4. ***Broad Food Selection:*** While the low FODMAP diet restricts certain types of carbohydrates, it still allows for a wide variety of foods to be consumed. This ensures that individuals can maintain a balanced and nutritious diet while managing their symptoms.

5. ***Evidence-Based***: The efficacy of the low FODMAP diet is supported by a growing body of scientific research. Numerous studies have demonstrated its effectiveness in reducing symptoms of IBS and other gastrointestinal disorders.

6. ***Reduction in Gut Inflammation***: Some research suggests that reducing FODMAP intake may help decrease inflammation in the gut, which can contribute to overall gut health and reduce symptoms associated with conditions like IBS.

7. ***Potential Weight Management:*** For some individuals, following a low FODMAP diet may lead to weight loss or weight management. This can be attributed to the elimination of high-calorie, high-FODMAP foods that may contribute to weight gain or exacerbate symptoms of bloating and discomfort.

8. ***Better Understanding of Food Sensitivities***: By identifying and avoiding specific FODMAP-containing

foods that trigger symptoms, individuals gain a better understanding of their own food sensitivities. This knowledge empowers them to make informed dietary choices that support their digestive health.

9. ***Long-Term Management Strategy***: While the low FODMAP diet is often used as a short-term intervention to identify trigger foods, some people may find that they can continue to follow a modified version of the diet long-term to manage their symptoms and prevent flare-ups.

10. ***Complementary to Other Therapies***: The low FODMAP diet can be used in conjunction with other therapies for IBS, such as medication, stress management, and dietary supplements.

This multi-faceted approach can provide comprehensive symptom relief and improve overall well-being.

It's important to note that the low FODMAP diet is not appropriate for everyone, and it should be undertaken with the guidance of a qualified healthcare professional, such as a registered dietitian, who can provide personalized advice and support. Additionally, while the low FODMAP diet can be highly effective for managing symptoms of IBS, it may not be necessary or beneficial for individuals without gastrointestinal issues

CHAPTER SEVEN

Low FODMAPS Benefits IBS

Irritable Bowel Syndrome (IBS) is a gastrointestinal disorder characterized by symptoms like abdominal pain, bloating, diarrhea, and constipation. One dietary approach gaining traction in managing IBS symptoms is the low FODMAP diet.

Fermentable Oligosaccharides, Disaccharides, Monosaccharides, and Polyols are a class of short-chain carbohydrates that the small intestine is not very good at absorbing. When they reach the colon, they ferment, leading to gas production and bloating in some individuals, particularly those with IBS.

To relieve symptoms, the low-FODMAPS diet calls for cutting back on or avoiding foods high in fructooligosaccharides. These foods include certain fruits (like apples, cherries, and watermelon), vegetables (such as onions, garlic, and cauliflower), legumes, wheat-based products, certain dairy products, and sweeteners like sorbitol and mannitol.

The connection between low FODMAPs and IBS lies in the fact that reducing FODMAP intake can help reduce symptoms such as bloating, gas, and abdominal pain in many individuals with IBS. Several studies have shown the efficacy of the low FODMAP diet in improving IBS symptoms, with some reporting symptom improvement in up to 75% of patients.

It's essential to note that the low FODMAP diet is not a one-size-fits-all solution. IBS is a complex condition with various triggers and symptoms, and what works for one person may not work for another. Additionally, the low FODMAP diet is typically recommended under the guidance of a healthcare professional, such as a registered dietitian, to ensure adequate nutrient intake and proper implementation.

While the low FODMAP diet can be effective in managing IBS symptoms, it's not intended as a long-term solution. The diet is typically implemented in phases, starting with a strict elimination phase where high-FODMAP foods are removed from the diet entirely, followed by a reintroduction phase to identify individual trigger foods, and finally, a maintenance phase where a more personalized diet is established.

In conclusion, the connection between low FODMAPs and IBS lies in the ability of reducing FODMAP intake to alleviate symptoms such as bloating, gas, and abdominal pain in many individuals with IBS. However, it's essential to approach the low FODMAP diet under the guidance of a healthcare professional to ensure effectiveness and safety.

CHAPTER EIGHT

Low FODMAPS Breakfast Recipes

The low FODMAP diet is designed to help manage symptoms of irritable bowel syndrome (IBS) by reducing intake of certain carbohydrates that are poorly absorbed in the small intestine. Breakfast is an important meal, and there are plenty of delicious and nutritious options available for those following a low FODMAP diet. Here are some ideas:

1. **Egg Muffins:** These are easy to make ahead of time and can be customized with various low FODMAP ingredients such as spinach, tomatoes, bell peppers, and lactose-free cheese.
2. ***Smoothies***: Use low FODMAP fruits like strawberries, blueberries, raspberries, or oranges as a base. Add lactose-free yogurt or almond milk, and

a handful of spinach or kale for added nutrients.

3. **_Quinoa Porridge_**: Cook quinoa in lactose-free milk or water, then top with low FODMAP fruits like banana or strawberries, and a sprinkle of nuts or seeds.

4. **_Omelet:_** Fill an omelet with low FODMAP ingredients like spinach, tomatoes, bell peppers, and a sprinkle of lactose-free cheese.

5. **_Overnight Oats_**: Mix oats with lactose-free milk or water, chia seeds, and a low FODMAP sweetener like maple syrup or a small amount of honey. Top with low FODMAP fruits like strawberries, kiwi, or blueberries.

6. **_Yogurt Parfait_**: Layer lactose-free yogurt with low FODMAP granola (made with oats, nuts, and seeds), and top with low FODMAP fruits like kiwi, strawberries, or blueberries.

7. **_Sourdough Toast_**: Enjoy a slice of toasted sourdough bread with toppings like peanut butter (made with just peanuts), mashed avocado, or lactose-free cream cheese. Add sliced tomatoes, cucumber, or smoked salmon for extra flavor.

8. ***Chia Seed Pudding***: Mix chia seeds with lactose-free milk, a low FODMAP sweetener, and a dash of vanilla extract. Let it sit in the fridge overnight to thicken, then top with low FODMAP fruits like raspberries, strawberries, or kiwi.
9. ***Buckwheat Pancakes***: Make pancakes using buckwheat flour, which is naturally low in FODMAPs. Serve with a drizzle of maple syrup and a side of low FODMAP fruits.
10. ***Tofu Scramble***: Sauteed tofu with spinach, tomatoes, and bell peppers for a flavorful and protein-packed breakfast option.

Remember to check portion sizes and ingredient lists to ensure they comply with the low FODMAP guidelines. Experiment with different combinations to find what works best for you, and consult with a dietitian for personalized advice.

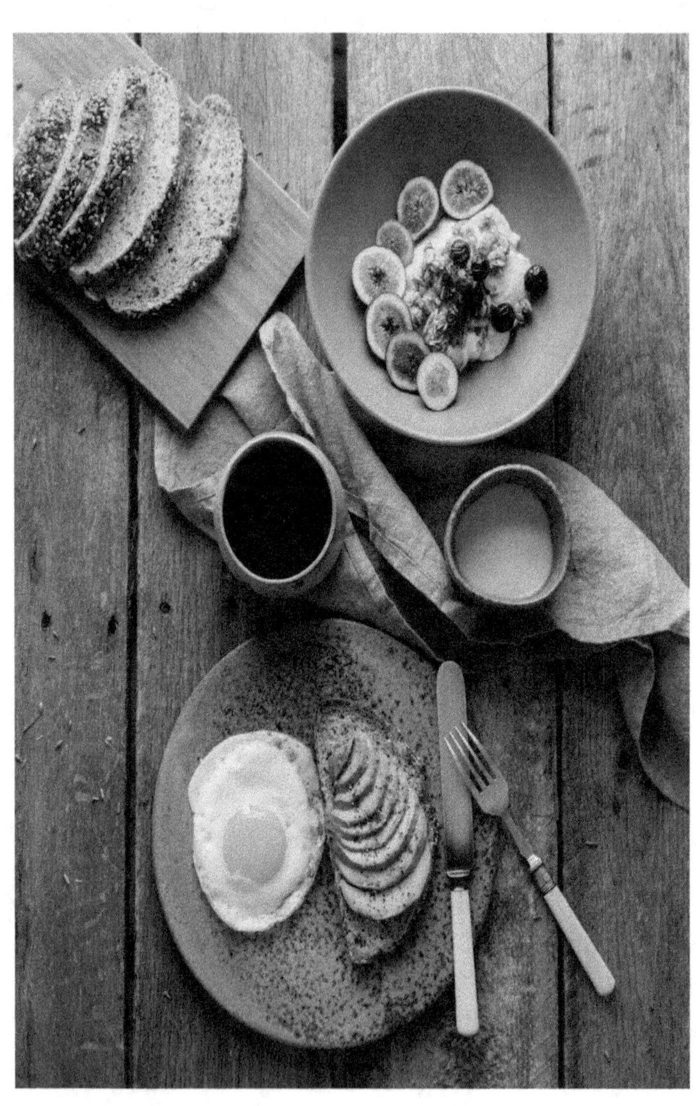

CHAPTER NINE

Lunch Break Dynamics

Lunch is more than just a meal; it's a significant pause in the day, offering nourishment and a chance to recharge both physically and mentally. It varies greatly across cultures, ranging from a quick bite on the go to a leisurely multi-course affair. Here's a comprehensive look at lunch:

1. ***Nutritional Importance:*** Lunch provides essential nutrients and energy to sustain productivity and mental alertness throughout the day. A balanced lunch should include carbohydrates for energy, protein for muscle repair and growth, healthy fats

for satiety, and a variety of vitamins and minerals for overall health.

2. ***Cultural Significance***: In many cultures, lunch is a social event. It's a time for family or colleagues to come together, share a meal, and connect. In some countries, like Spain, lunch is the largest meal of the day and can last for hours, while in others, like the United States, it's often a shorter break during the workday.

3. ***Types of Lunches***: Lunches can vary widely depending on factors such as cultural traditions, personal preferences, and dietary restrictions. Some common types include:

    - Quick and Portable: Sandwiches, salads, wraps, and other

grab-and-go options are popular for those with busy schedules.

- Home-cooked Meals: Many people prefer to prepare and bring their own lunch from home, which allows for greater control over ingredients and portion sizes.

- Restaurant or Takeout: Dining out for lunch is a convenient option for those who prefer not to cook or want to enjoy a meal with friends or colleagues.

- Street Food: In urban areas, street food vendors offer a wide range of lunch options, from falafel and tacos to noodles and kebabs.

4. ***Health Considerations***: While lunch can be an opportunity to indulge in tasty treats, it's important to make nutritious choices to support overall well-being. Incorporating fruits, vegetables, whole grains, and lean proteins into your lunch can help maintain a healthy diet and prevent energy crashes later in the day.

5. ***Workplace Dynamics:*** Lunch breaks can impact workplace culture and dynamics. Some companies encourage employees to take regular breaks and socialize over lunch, believing it fosters teamwork and creativity. Others may have a more fast-paced environment where employees eat at their desks or take shorter breaks to maximize productivity.

6. ***Environmental Impact:*** The choices we make for lunch, such as opting for plant-based meals or reducing food waste, can have significant environmental implications. Choosing locally sourced ingredients and minimizing single-use packaging can help reduce our carbon footprint.

In conclusion, lunch is not just a midday meal; it's a time to refuel, connect, and make conscious choices that support our health and well-being, as well as the health of the planet. Whether it's a simple sandwich at your desk or a lavish feast with friends, lunch plays a vital role in our daily lives.

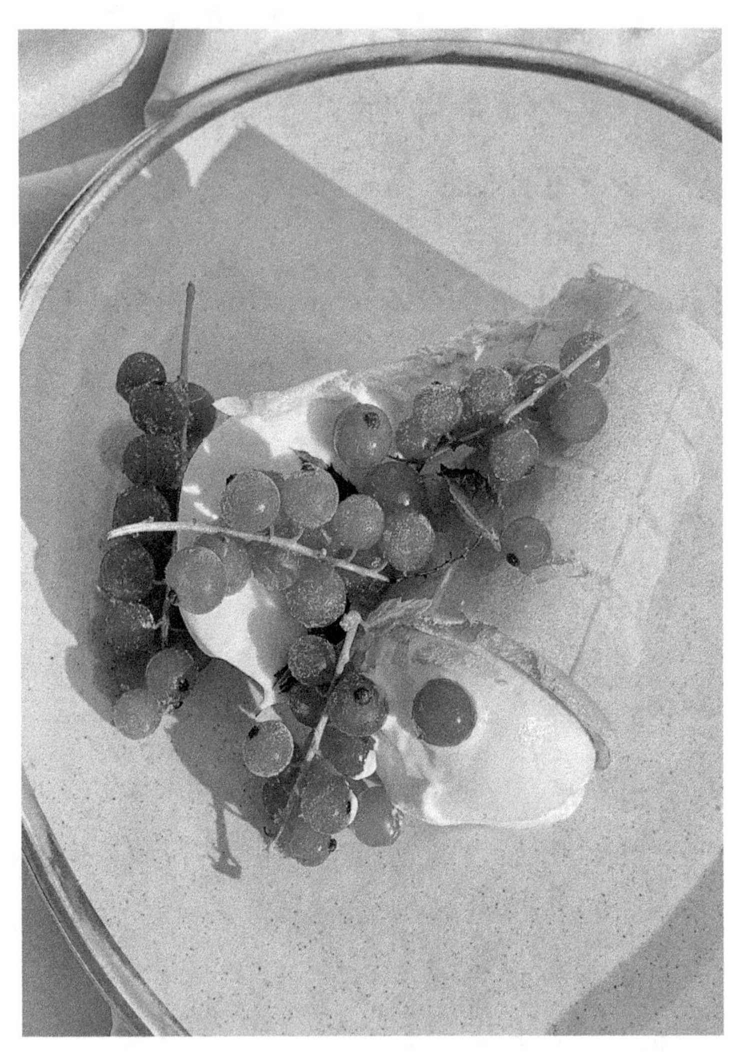

CHAPTER TEN

Low FODMAPS Dinner Recipes

Low FODMAP dinner recipes are designed to minimize foods containing certain types of carbohydrates that can cause digestive discomfort in some individuals, particularly those with irritable bowel syndrome (IBS) or other digestive issues. FODMAPs are fermentable oligosaccharides, disaccharides, monosaccharides, and polyols – types of carbohydrates that can ferment in the gut and lead to symptoms like bloating, gas, and abdominal pain.

Here are some comprehensive low FODMAP dinner recipes:

1. ***Grilled Chicken with Quinoa and Roasted Vegetables***:

   - Marinate chicken breasts in olive oil, lemon juice, garlic-infused oil, and herbs.

   - Cook quinoa separately according to package instructions.

   - Roast low FODMAP vegetables like zucchini, bell peppers, and carrots with a drizzle of olive oil, salt, and pepper.

   - Serve grilled chicken over cooked quinoa alongside roasted vegetables.

2. ***Salmon with Steamed Green Beans and Mashed Potatoes***:

   - Add salt, pepper, and lemon zest to salmon filets for seasoning.

- Salmon should be cooked through when baked or grilled.
- Steam green beans until tender.
- Boil potatoes until soft, then mash with lactose-free milk, butter, and chives.
- Serve salmon with steamed green beans and mashed potatoes.

3. Low FODMAP Taco Bowl:

- Cook ground turkey or beef with taco seasoning (check for low FODMAP ingredients or make your own blend).
- Prepare a base of cooked rice or quinoa.
- Top with cooked meat, shredded lettuce, diced tomatoes, sliced olives, and lactose-free cheese.

- Add a dollop of lactose-free sour cream and a squeeze of lime juice.

4. ***Stir-Fried Shrimp with Rice Noodles and Vegetables***:

   - Stir-fry shrimp with low FODMAP vegetables like bell peppers, bok choy, and carrots in a garlic-infused oil.
   - Cook rice noodles according to package instructions.
   - Toss cooked noodles with stir-fried shrimp and vegetables.
   - Garnish with chopped scallions (green parts only) and a sprinkle of sesame seeds.

5. ***Grilled Steak with Baked Potatoes and Asparagus:***

- Marinate steak in a mixture of olive oil, Worcestershire sauce (check for no onion or garlic), and herbs.
- Bake potatoes until tender.
- Grill steak to desired doneness.
- Roast asparagus with olive oil, salt, and pepper until crisp-tender.
- Serve grilled steak with baked potatoes and asparagus.

Remember to tailor recipes to your specific dietary needs and preferences, and always check ingredient labels for hidden sources of FODMAPs. Additionally, portion sizes and individual tolerance levels may vary, so it's essential to listen to your body and adjust as

needed.

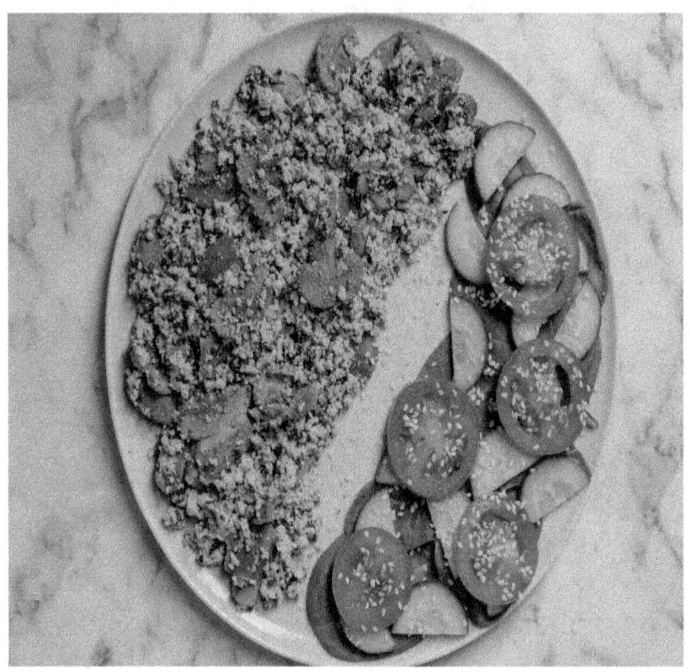

CHAPTER ELEVEN

Snack Recipes Ideas

Snack recipes are versatile and can range from savory to sweet, catering to various tastes and occasions. Here's a comprehensive overview covering different types of snack recipes:

1. *Savory Snacks:*

    - Vegetable Platter: Arrange sliced cucumbers, carrots, bell peppers, and cherry tomatoes on a platter. Accompany with ranch dressing or hummus for dunkling.

    - Stuffed Mushrooms: Stuff mushroom caps with a blend of breadcrumbs, cream cheese, garlic, and herbs. Bake until golden brown.

- o Mini Quiches: Make bite-sized quiches by filling mini muffin tins with a mixture of eggs, cheese, vegetables, and bacon or ham.
- o Samosas: These triangular pastries filled with spiced potatoes, peas, and sometimes meat are popular in many cuisines, especially Indian and Middle Eastern.
- o Spinach and Feta Puffs: Fill puff pastry squares with a mixture of spinach, feta cheese, and garlic. Bake until golden and crispy.
- o Buffalo Cauliflower Bites: Coat cauliflower florets in a spicy buffalo sauce and bake until

crispy. Serve with ranch dressing for dipping.

2. **_Sweet Snacks:_**

   o Fruit Skewers: Thread chunks of pineapple, strawberries, grapes, and melon onto skewers for a colorful and refreshing snack.

   o Chocolate Covered Pretzels: Dip pretzel rods or twists into melted chocolate and sprinkle with toppings like crushed nuts, sprinkles, or sea salt.

   o Energy Bites: Mix together oats, nut butter, honey, and add-ins like chocolate chips, dried fruit, or seeds. Roll into bite-sized balls and refrigerate until firm.

   o Banana Sushi: Spread peanut butter or Nutella on a banana, then roll it in granola or crushed cereal. Slice into bite-sized pieces.

- Cinnamon Sugar Pita Chips: Brush pita bread with melted butter, sprinkle with cinnamon sugar, and bake until crisp. Serve with fruit salsa or yogurt dip.

- Mini Cheesecakes: Make individual cheesecakes in a muffin tin. Top with fruit compote, chocolate sauce, or whipped cream.

3. ***Healthy Snacks***:

- Greek Yogurt Parfait: Layer Greek yogurt with granola, berries, and a drizzle of honey for a nutritious and satisfying snack.

- Edamame: Steam edamame and toss with sea salt for a protein-packed snack that's perfect for munching on the go.

- Roasted Chickpeas: Toss chickpeas with olive oil and your favorite spices, then roast until crispy. They make a crunchy and satisfying snack.

- Apple Nachos: Slice apples and arrange them on a plate. Drizzle with almond butter or peanut butter and sprinkle with toppings like granola, coconut flakes, and chocolate chips.

- Trail Mix: Combine nuts, seeds, dried fruit, and a sprinkle of dark chocolate chips for a portable

and nutritious snack that's perfect
for hiking or road trips.

Snack recipes offer endless possibilities for creativity and customization, making them perfect for satisfying cravings and fueling busy days. Whether you're in the mood for something savory, sweet, or healthy, there's a snack recipe out there to suit your tastes.

CHAPTER TWELVE

Dessert Recipes Overview

Dessert recipes offer a delightful finale to any meal, ranging from simple classics to elaborate creations. Here's a comprehensive overview covering various types of desserts:

1. ***Cakes and Cupcakes***: From traditional sponge cakes to rich chocolate cakes, this category offers endless possibilities. Classic flavors like vanilla, chocolate, and red velvet are always popular, but you can also experiment with unique combinations like carrot cake or lemon-blueberry. Cupcakes offer individual portions and can be decorated

creatively with frosting, sprinkles, or fondant.

2. ***Pies and Tarts:*** Pies come in many forms, including fruit pies (e.g., apple, cherry), custard pies (e.g., pumpkin, key lime), and cream pies (e.g., chocolate cream, coconut cream). Tarts are similar but often have a thinner crust and can feature various fillings like fruit compotes, custards, or chocolate ganache.

3. ***Cookies and Bars:*** Cookies range from soft and chewy to crisp and crunchy, with flavors like chocolate chip, oatmeal raisin, and sugar cookies being perennial favorites. Bars can include brownies, blondies, and layered treats like Nanaimo bars, offering a convenient way to serve desserts for gatherings.

4. ***Puddings and Custards***: Creamy and comforting, puddings and custards come in many flavors and textures. Classic examples include rice pudding, bread pudding, crème brûlée, and flan. These desserts are often made with eggs, milk, sugar, and flavorings like vanilla, chocolate, or caramel.

5. ***Ice Cream and Frozen Treats:*** Homemade ice cream allows for endless flavor combinations, from traditional vanilla and chocolate to more adventurous options like pistachio-honey or salted caramel. Other frozen treats include sorbets, gelatos, and popsicles, which can be made with fresh fruit purees or juices.

6. ***Pastries and Danishes:*** Pastries encompass a wide range of desserts,

including croissants, éclairs, and cream puffs. Danishes are a type of pastry typically filled with fruit, cheese, or custard and topped with icing or glaze. These treats require some skill to master but are well worth the effort.

7. ***Trifles and Parfaits:*** Trifles are layered desserts usually consisting of cake, custard, fruit, and whipped cream. Parfaits follow a similar concept but can incorporate ingredients like yogurt, granola, nuts, and berries, offering a lighter option with endless variations.

8. ***Specialty Desserts***: This category includes desserts with unique cultural or regional significance, such as tiramisu from Italy, baklava from the Middle East, or mochi from Japan. These desserts often feature distinct ingredients and

preparation methods, adding a global flair to your culinary repertoire.

When creating dessert recipes, consider factors like dietary restrictions (e.g., gluten-free, vegan), seasonal ingredients, and presentation aesthetics. Experimenting with flavors, textures, and techniques allows for endless creativity in the world of dessert-making. Whether you're baking for a special occasion or simply indulging your sweet tooth, there's a dessert recipe out there to satisfy every craving.

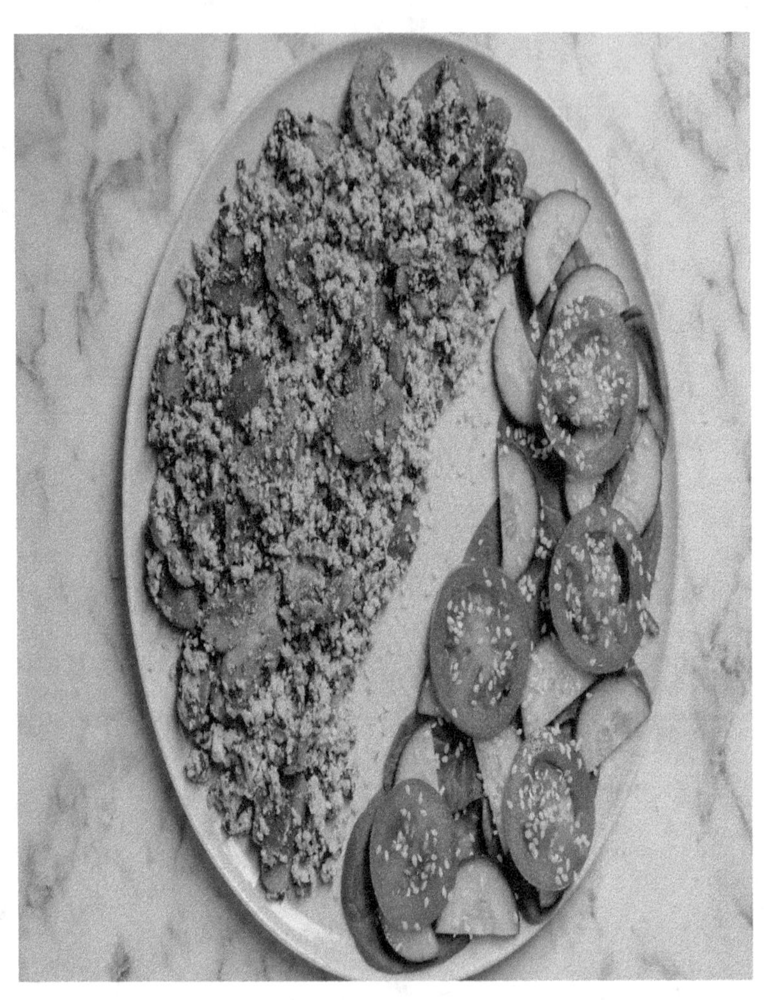

CONCLUSION

In crafting this low FODMAPs diet cookbook, our primary aim has been to empower individuals managing digestive discomfort to embrace a fulfilling culinary journey without compromising taste or health. Through a meticulous curation of recipes, we've endeavored to demonstrate that adhering to a low FODMAPs diet doesn't equate to deprivation, but rather an opportunity to explore an array of flavorful, nourishing dishes. By offering a diverse selection of breakfasts, lunches, dinners, snacks, and desserts, we've sought to cater to every palate and occasion, ensuring that no matter the dietary restrictions, there's always a delicious option at hand. Moreover, we've strived to foster a sense of creativity and adaptability, encouraging readers to experiment with ingredients, flavors, and cooking techniques, thus empowering them to customize recipes to suit their individual preferences and nutritional needs. Ultimately, this cookbook serves as a testament to the transformative power of mindful eating, demonstrating that by making informed dietary choices, individuals can not only alleviate digestive discomfort but also cultivate a deeper appreciation for the joys of cooking and sharing wholesome meals with loved ones. As you embark on your culinary journey, may this cookbook serve as a trusted companion, inspiring you to savor each moment and relish in the nourishment that comes from honoring your body's unique needs.

www.ingramcontent.com/pod-product-compliance
Lightning Source LLC
Chambersburg PA
CBHW051840250726
48659CB00005B/1938